Weight Loss

The Obstacles in Weight Loss and How to Overcome Them

Table of Contents

Introduction

There are many problems associated with being overweight. Many time's people do not realize that they are overweight. Hence, they remain oblivious to the damage that is caused by it. Being overweight can lead to several life threatening diseases.

Our lifestyle and our diet have a lot to say about our overall health. This is especially true for people in their middle age. For people who have a stressful and hectic routine without any time for sleep and eat proper meals, being overweight becomes a definite possibility. On the other hand, people who make smart decisions and take some time out for themselves every day reap the rewards eventually.

We rarely feel the effects of time on our body. Until one day we realize how things have changed. You look back and think about the days you used to be in the school's soccer team but now you find yourself gasping for breath just by climbing a few stairs. This is something that everyone has to go through and something that is unavoidable. Through the course of this article, we will discuss some of the strategies that you can employ to delay the aforementioned effects as much as possible. With proper diet and regular exercise, you can stay fit longer and hopefully enjoy your life without any dependencies.

SECTION I

Reasons for weight gain

The human body is a machine and like any other machine, as time passes, it wears and tears more over time and becomes more prone to problems. Of the many problems that accompany aging, one of the key problems is weight gain. Weight gain is a severe area of concern because it is not only a problem in itself but it leads to several other health issues. Not only that but it can also lead to low self-esteem in people who are generally more conscious about their physical appearance etc. Even if we ignore for the time being the aesthetic concerns that may arise there are many health concerns that will arise like high blood pressure, heart disease, joint pain etc.

Dietary Imbalance

Weight gain is something that can be easily controlled in youth but as you get older you don't have the same agility and stamina in you to burn the extra calories and keep yourself fit. So, a possible solution is to control the causes that may in the first place lead to weight gain. Different theorists have different explanations for weight gain in old age, but a quite significant and common reason which they all identify is dietary imbalance. Although dietary imbalance is not age specific its effects become more severe as you grow older. People generally end up getting more weight because they do not take care of their diet. They usually end up taking in more carbs and fats and less fibers to digest them which in turn causes them to gain more weight.

A simple remedy can be for you to start taking in a balanced diet. That way you will be more likely to avoid this problem of weight gain and the associated problems. Another reason which is quite common in elder people is lack of mobility and physical exercise. This may be the result of a physical condition like arthritis. As a result people further restrict their mobility, ignoring the fact that a possible reason for this could be their excessive weight in the first place, which can be solved through light exercises. But people generally end up becoming more flaccid, and cause their condition to get worse, causing further weight gain and consequently more joint pains, and the loop goes on.

Diabetes

Even if people are not encountering any of these problems, they may generally become less motivated and lazier with growing age. However, this is not the only reason. There may be some other health issues that can lead to weight gain. As you approach fifty, people will sometimes end up getting severe diseases and a common one is diabetes. Diabetes causes your body to stop producing insulin and external insulin has to be injected to keep the blood sugar level in control. People who use insulin usually have to take up a meal that is equivalent to the amount injected to prevent them from suffering from a low blood sugar level, known as Hypoglycemia. What happens consequently is that the body ends up taking more amount of sugar than it actually requires and this extra amount of calories intake by the body can lead to weight gain. There are two ways of avoiding this issue.

If you do develop this disease keep a stern check on the amount of sugar you are taking and control it to a point where you don't have to take external insulin. If people let things go as they are, then they will end up taking insulin to counter those extra sugar meals, which consequently will lead to weight gain and the health issues will keep on propagating.

Stress

Another reason for weight gain that people generally overlook is stress. There was a study conducted in which it was found that people who live in less stressful environments and have a good job, a happy family and so on, are less prone to diseases and weight gain. Stress in itself is a psychological disease which causes a hormone to be released in your body generally termed as the stress hormone. This causes an increase in appetite and to counter it you turn towards your comfort foods. People generally increase the intake of high calorie fast foods and high caffeine sodas to keep themselves distracted and to alleviate their stress. In the process they end up taking in heavy amounts of calories, which can significantly increase their weight. As people get older, their responsibilities increase and they end up getting more stressed out. They no longer have the physical strength to work more or put in more effort and they end up getting more stressed out which in turn leads to more weight gain.

Especially when people start hitting the age of fifty, they start realizing that they have fewer years left in them to work and if they think that they have not achieved the goals they had set for themselves, they may start overexerting themselves. They may become sleep deprived and more tired and that can in fact lead to more weight gain. A study was conducted that showed people who sleep for around eight to nine hours a day were less prone to weight gain whereas those who slept for only five to six hours gained more weight. There are many possible explanations but a common one that is generally given is that sleep deprived people might feel more tired. To keep themselves active they may seek high calorie snacks like chocolates to keep their energy levels up during the day and this excess calorie intake turns out to be the reason they end up getting overweight.

Hormonal Changes

Elderly women may become more prone to weight gain as they reach menopause. Studies show that menopause can cause women to gain more weight especially around their abdomen which is usually referred to as bloating of the abdomen. This may be due to the hormonal changes that are accompanied with menopause or this may be due to the fact that the body becomes more water retentive which in severe cases can take the form of edema. As the body starts retaining more fluids, parts of the body can start becoming swollen and this can in turn lead to more weight gain.

There may be several other possible explanations for weight gain. It may be due to some other diseases like underactive thyroid gland which consequently is slowing down the body's metabolism and causing the body to gain more weight. Other than that there are many other psychological and physiological explanations for weight gain but the above mentioned ones are the most noticeable. None of the problems are such that they are unavoidable. They can all be avoided; all that is needed is just a little bit of effort and a little bit of care. If people realize how weight gain can deteriorate their physical condition and compare it to the effort that is needed to avoid weight gain, they would never be careless in this matter, ever.

SECTION II

Diet Solutions

Losing weight requires work on two major fronts. One, you need to make sure that you take some time out of your daily routine to indulge in some physical activities. And number two, you need to alter your diet plan. Consuming a low calorie diet devoid of any fats can prove to be quite helpful in shedding some pounds. Having said that, let us now look at some of the foods that are known to be quite helpful in losing weight. Because of this property, they are also known as 'super foods.'

Superfoods

Almonds

Almonds are an excellent option if you are looking to get back into shape and get a flat belly. Almonds have many properties that make them so useful as a source of food and energy. Although they have a high calorie content, almonds can help you lose weight fast. They are also a good source of Vitamin E and protein. We all know that by consuming ample amount of vitamin E, we can repair the damaged skin cells which leaves our skin feeling fresh and revitalized. Also, almonds can help in fighting the loss of muscle mass because they are a good source of protein.

Leafy Greens

Second on our list are the leafy greens. They are nature's best detox agents. Over a certain period of time, our body accumulates unwanted substances that are by products of some of the chemical reactions that take place in our body. These can be toxins for the body in more than one way and need to be removed. Leafy greens, especially kale and spinach, are excellent detox agents that will clear your body of all toxins. These leafy vegetables also contain high fiber content which is crucial in maintaining healthy motility in the alimentary canal. Leafy greens have very low calorie content, therefore they are very helpful in losing weight and should be included in our daily diets.

Oats

Oats are another amazing food choice on our list that can prove to be really helpful in losing weight. There are two main advantages of consuming oats. Number one is that oats can be a steady source of energy throughout the day. They have a low calorie content but if you eat oatmeal for breakfast, you'll not have to fight the urge of stuffing yourself with more food as you will already feel full. And number two, oats help the body in keeping the level of cholesterol in check. Hence this is the highly recommended food for keeping most heart related problems at bay.

Olive Oil

When we say to avoid fats we mean to avoid certain types of fats. This is because there are certain types of fats that contribute to weight gain. Whereas there are certain type of fats such as the poly un-saturated fats contained in olive oil which can in fact help in reducing the fat content of the body. By substituting the cooking oil in our homes with olive oil, we can ensure that the household gets a healthy amount of oleic acid in their system. Oleic acid is a naturally found compound in olive oil that is known to help in the breakdown of excess fats in the body. Hence, olive oil can help you and your family get back in shape. Due to its low cholesterol content, olive oil is often recommended for heart patients as well.

Beans

Just like all the food sources discussed above, beans can also prove to be a great ally if weight loss is on your agenda. The best thing about beans is that they are a slow-energy releasing food. What this means is that beans constantly supply energy to the body, up till many hours after their consumption. This can help fight your hunger pangs as the digestive system will indicate to the brain that there is enough stockpile of useable energy available and hence there is no need to eat more. In addition to that, beans are also an excellent source of vital minerals that are crucial for proper functioning of the body.

Peppermint

For those of us who are somewhat familiar with herbal medicine, peppermint has been used for a long time as a healing agent. However, another brilliant property of peppermint is that it can help your digestive system as well. This will help quell the sudden urges for food and like the aforementioned leafy vegetable, peppermint is also an excellent detox agent. Drinking three to four cups of peppermint tea everyday will not only help you in losing weight but will also leave your skin with a delightful glow as your innards are cleared of all the piled up toxins.

Green Tea

One of the most well-known slimming agents in the world is green tea. Green tea can be used to target the fat deposits in troublesome areas of the body. For example, the bloating around the abdomen can be quite stubborn and burning this fat might be a bit of a challenge. Thankfully, by drinking green tea daily we can address this problem to a significant degree. We already know that when we are over the fifty year mark, our metabolism rate loses much of its potency. Hence the ingested food is no longer digested properly. Green tea can help improve your body's metabolism rate so that you can stay fit and healthy all day long.

Kelp

Seaweed can also be used to aid in weight loss in the elderly. As the years go by, our thyroid glands fail to produce the required amount of hormones. As a result, the state of 'hypothyroidism' exists within the body. With the onset of hypothyroidism, the basal metabolism rate of the body suffers a great deal. Seaweeds like kelp in particular are a rich source of iodine. This iodine can be used in the production of thyroid hormones so that your metabolism rate is regulated. Other than that, kelp also contains some minerals that can aid in breaking down the stubborn fats inside the body.

Apple Cider Vinegar

If you are looking to 'service' you alimentary canal, adding apple cider vinegar to your daily diet will enable you to achieve that. Having detox properties, this vinegar is an excellent tonic against the stubborn bacteria that reside inside our digestive system. These bacteria can hinder the proper digestion of food and often produce many toxins as byproducts. As the efficiency of the digestive system is reduced, food is not properly broken down. Using apple cider vinegar you can counteract this problem and lose some weight because it aids in the breakdown of fat deposits inside the body.

Cranberry Juice

This is another liquid diet that has shown positive results in people looking to lose weight. Drinking a glass of cranberry juice will supply your body with much needed energy to carry you around thus quelling the hunger pangs. Other than that it is also a rich source of Vitamin C. Like other such fluids, cranberry juice is also very beneficial for the urinary system of the body. By ensuring removal of excess fluids and proper water retention, the body is able to burn off fats faster and more effectively.

Asparagus

Asparagus is a vegetable that has numerous beneficial properties for the elderly. It is a rich source of minerals such as zinc and potassium. This low calorie – high fiber vegetable is an excellent substitute for your mid-day snacks. It also provides the body with a much needed dose of vitamins. Because of the dietary fibers, the motility (of the alimentary canal) remains on a healthy level. This increases the metabolism rate which ensures that you feel energetic all day to go out and about. Eventually, you need energy in order to carry out the physical exertions required to lose weight. Other than that, asparagus has also been known to treat the inflammations and rheumatism. Thus it should be a must in your daily diet if you are looking to live healthy.

Tomatoes

Tomatoes can go a long way to solving the weight loss issue. Due to hormonal imbalance in the body, the concentration of ghrelin inside the body increases whereas the concentration of leptin decreases. Ghrelin is the hormone which instigates hunger whereas leptin quells it. Due to several stressors like inadequate sleep for example, the balance between these two hormones is disturbed. There is a sudden increase in ghrelin concentration whereas the levels of leptin drop. In order to remedy this situation, tomatoes can help reverse the leptin resistance that develops in the body. This helps regulate the body's basal metabolism rate which aids in weight loss.

Garlic

Many people have their reservations regarding the use of garlic because of the bad breath that follows as a result. However, trust me when I say this, the bad breath is but a small price to pay in comparison to all the benefits that come with using garlic. Garlic is a member of the onion family. The biggest advantage of using garlic is that it contains a compound named allicin. This compound plays a significant role in fighting the bacteria inside our body especially those residing inside the digestive tract. This results in a healthier digestive system which is more important than you realize if you truly want to lose some weight.

Goji Berry

Goji Berry or wolfberry as it is also known is a bright red berry that can be found in many of the Asian and European countries. Goji berries are often referred to as a 'super-food' because of the potency in helping people lose weight. These berries are either eaten as fresh or they can also be used in the dried form. However, the best way to consume goji berries is in the form of juices and shakes. There are many nutritional supplements in the market that have goji berries as one of their core ingredients.

There are many advantages of eating the wolfberry. However, the biggest advantage as we stated earlier is that goji berries help in losing weight. These berries have a very low calorie content yet deliver a healthy dose of vitamins and minerals. Their anti-oxidant properties can also help in removing the free radicals inside the body that are produced as byproducts. Eliminating the free radicals is important because they have been known to cause potential life-threating diseases such as artery clogging plaque as well as cancer.

Hemp seeds are derived from the hemp plant and are an excellent source of protein. This makes them ideal for consumption, especially for mature women who have to make up for the loss of muscle mass. Other than that, hemp seeds also contain fiber, vitamins, enzymes and essential amino acids. Because of the high protein content, hemp seeds can help in quelling hunger pangs throughout the day. This allows you to skip a meal allowing you to embark upon an intensive diet routine.

The hemp plant can grow almost anywhere in the world. The plant also blossoms quickly (within 2 to 3 months). This makes hemp seeds an affordable and readily available source of food. The best way to consume hemp seeds is to sprinkle a spoon or two on your cereal. You can also use it with yoghurt for breakfast. Hemp seed milk is a very good alternative to dairy milk as it contains very few calories.

Baobab

The Baobab fruit is often touted as a 'super-fruit' because of its ability to aid in weight loss. This is because the baobab fruit contains up to 50% fiber of which 66% can be soluble. The soluble fiber is an important source of energy for the body. Insoluble fiber is the kind that cannot be utilized by the body but is important for the motility of the digestive tract. However, there are certain bacteria present inside the intestines that can break down the soluble facts. This process is known as the prebiotic effect.

Among the soluble fats, pectin is one that has high viscosity. The soluble fiber found in the Baobab fruit is mainly composed of pectin. This gel-like substance makes you feel sated for long. Pectin increases the time taken by the food in the stomach to pass into the intestine. Hence, by increasing your consumption of Baobab fruit, you can feel sated for longer allowing you to follow the required dieting plan with ease.

Flaxseeds

Flax seeds, also referred to as linseeds are one of the richest sources of Omega 3 fatty acids. These fatty acids are very beneficial to health. These seeds are very low in carbohydrates and very rich in dietary fibers. Being low in carbs and rich in fibers allows these seeds to be a great recipe for weight loss. Fibers help in forming bulk in the stomach and makes the digestion process easier. Having high amounts of both soluble and insoluble fiber allows them to help in the detoxification of the intestines and because of this they are very healthy and beneficial especially from someone aiming for weight loss.

These seeds are rich in good fats so it provides a healthier diet. Moreover being high in fibers allows you to not feel hunger pangs for a longer period of time. Since these seeds are forming bulk and not causing hunger pangs it can lead to greater gaps in between your meals, which allows you to eat less and as a result achieve weight loss. Although it has fats in it, mostly omega 3, these fats are not saturated and so they will not accumulate in your body and cause weight gain. These are low cholesterol good fats that are easily water soluble and very beneficial for your body. Many nutritionists would encourage you to make flax seeds a part of your everyday meals if you aim to achieve weight gain in a lesser amount of time.

The final entry on our list in this book is wheatgrass. Like Baobab fruit, the wheatgrass contains a healthy amount of minerals, amino acids and enzymes. Consuming wheatgrass will not only suppress your hunger but will also revitalize your body's metabolic rate. This will help you burn all the extra calories and lose some weight. Other than weight loss, wheat grass can also help in full body detox.

The most common way to consome wheatgrass is in the form of smoothies and juices. It is also sometimes used in powdered form because this way we can enjoy the best of its nutritional value. Wheatgrass is also a rich source of Vitamins A, C, K and B.

There are several other nuts, fruits and vegetables such as chilies, bananas, walnuts, melons and so on that are an excellent choice if weight loss is your objective. However, it is important to realize that you need to be patient with the results. Many times, people resort to crash dieting as they try to instantly lose weight. As a consequence they suddenly stop eating altogether and start eating only fluids such as tea and juice. Although this may produce some results, they would often be a temporary fix.

The human body adapts with the changes around it. Thus when we suddenly stop eating altogether, the body goes into starvation mode. In the starvation mode, the body makes changes so that minimum amount of energy reserves inside the body is utilized. Hence, even though we have restricted our diets we often do not see any considerable changes taking place because our body becomes used to the lack of food.

In order to counter this, experts suggest to avoid crash dieting and to adopt a more gentle approach. Be sporadic. Don't let your body adapt to the new changes. That is the only way you can actually lose weight without the fear of it reappearing any time soon. However, this does not mean that you can ease up on your exercise and diet routine. Constant effort is required from your side in order to maintain a healthy lifestyle.

SECTION III

Exercise Solutions

Being vigilant about what to eat and what not to is a good practice. However, it is of no use if we do not reaffirm this strategy with proper exercise. In the end, you need to sweat and make an effort if you truly want to lose weight. Dieting alone is not enough to do the job. There are many easy exercises that we can use to achieve our weight goal. Let us now look at some of the most effective ones.

Aerobic Exercises

Walking/Running

Aerobic exercises are by far the most effective way of burning fat. Walking or running is by far the easiest exercises to perform. The best thing about such aerobic exercises is that you need very little investment to get you started. Also you are not bound by any time frame and you can go whenever you want. All you need is a pair of good running shoes and you are all set. When running, try not to run too fast as you will be out of breath pretty soon. Try to maintain a steady pace. To analyze your speed, check if you are able to say 2-3 sentences easily while running. If you find yourself gasping for breath, you are going too fast and you need to adjust accordingly. Also it might be a good idea to time your runs. Start by a warm up walk for five minutes and then jog for one minute. In between these jogs, take one minute walking breaks. Using this strategy will enable you to complete thirty minutes of workout even if you have never run before in your life. You only need to run four days a week. With the passage of time you can increase the intensity of this exercise by increasing the minutes you run and taking shorter breaks in between. Just half an hour run can help you burn as much as 300 calories!

Cardiovascular Exercises

Swimming

Walking and running are good exercises to start off with. However, these exercises cannot bring your weight down overnight. You need to stay focused and determined. On the other hand, if you are looking to step it up a notch and really burn some calories then swimming is the right choice. Swimming is considered the best form of cardio and it has numerous benefits. Not only will it help you lose weight but swimming is also the best option if you are looking to relax and beat the summer heat. You may not realize it but swimming for an hour or so can help you burn up to 600 calories! This is twice as much as what you can achieve by running. However, for most of you ladies over 50, swimming at a stretch for an hour might not be possible. So, like running, we divide our swimming hour into sets. For starters, a ten minutes swim followed by a five minutes rest would be ideal to get you going. Once you develop the stamina for it, you can increase the intensity. Swimming is a full body exercise that can help you to get rid of excess fat fast.

Cycling

Cycling is also a great cardio exercise. Like running, this too requires little investment and you are not time bound. For swimming, unless you have a pool at your house, you need to adjust your schedule according to the timings of the pool. However, if you own a cycle, you can be on your way whenever you want. If you think that your schedules are too tight and that you will not be able to take some time out for exercising then there is one thing that will definitely work.

Start going to your office on your bicycles instead of cars. Leave home ten minutes early. By cycling for one hour a day you can burn around 600 – 800 calories a day. Also, it is not important to ride the bicycle with high intensity. Elderly women can benefit a lot simply from light cycling. Like in the case of the aforementioned exercises, it is not necessary to complete the whole routine in one go. You can break it up in sets and allow yourself some time to recuperate. It is important not to push your body too far as you will end up doing more harm than good.

Strength Training

With the passage of time, our body loses much of its muscle mass. This is especially prevalent when we are past our middle age. The lost mass is replaced as fat which can lead to overall weight gain. Strength Training Exercises can go a long way to reclaiming the lost muscle mass. However, before we proceed further it is important to remind you that your body has its limitations. It is not as forgiving as it was when you were twenty years old. Stretching your body past its breaking point will make you regret your decisions in the first place. Hence, before indulging in any exercises particularly when you are past the 50 year mark, it is important to have a full body check up. You know what they say, better safe than sorry.

The best thing to do is to discuss your physical condition with a doctor and find out whether you are allowed to perform certain exercises or not. Generally, when you indulge in strength training exercises (for older people) your aim is not the weight but the number of reps that you do. Your aim is not to gain mass but to maintain what is necessary to be healthy.

Strength training exercises are also an easy way to reduce weight. These too don't require much investment. Just a couple of dumbbells and a comfortable bend will do the trick. Try to start off slow and work with different muscles of the body. Don't focus on one part alone. Do mixed exercises that focus on the biceps, triceps, wings, and chest and shoulder muscles. Arm curls and arm raises are two excellent exercises to get you started. Do not worry about the cramps. You are bound to get them at the start. But if you stick to your routine you will start to feel comfortable and energized within a weeks' time.

Some people are not so comfortable in using weights. There are a variety of exercises that do not require any weights at all and can be performed easily at home. Squats, jumping jacks, planks, pushups and crunches are all very good exercises that focus on different parts of the body. There are many seven minute workout routines available on the internet. You can check out the videos on YouTube.

In choosing your exercise you must keep in mind your physical and age constraints and must not try to overexert yourself, because that may in turn prove to be more harmful to you in the long run.